Contents

LOVE, LIES AND LIPSTICK

By
Laurie Shoemaker

CHAPTER ONE

Studying beauty techniques over the centuries is an interesting pastime. I remember my Southern Belle mother telling me that my grandmother took baths in milk and honey to keep her skin unblemished. Yuk. It might work, but you would have to have a second bath to rinse all the residue off! Honey was also used as a moisturizer as well as turmeric oil.

Apple cider vinegar was cherished as a rinse for the hair. Turmeric, honey and castor oil were used as a face mask to perk up skin. Splashing ice water was a daily trick. Women thought it "woke up skin" so they plunged their faces in a bowl of freezing water each morning. Castor oil was also used to achieve lush eyelashes.

Old time beauty regimes were correct in one area. Almost every lady cleansed her face at night with Pond's facial cream. It removed makeup but left a definite slippery feeling afterward. So rose water was used as a toner to clarify the skin.

Some of these remedies are the basis for our fine cosmetics today. Let's discover in this little book the do's and don'ts of today's beauty routines. What products are best for your type of skin? What works and what doesn't? And lastly, what is it like to work in a cosmetic department?

I was a practicing makeup artist for twenty years and, from what I experience today, the products and techniques have improved and focus more on treating the elements of aging skin. Trends come and go; one year the 'look' will be heavy eye makeup and pale lips. The next year, lipstick is back with a bang and eyes are softer.

If you're a 'girly' girl who loves to spend time at makeup counters, or a career woman who wants a fast and easy way to look professional, this book is for you. And for those 'beauties of a certain age,' you will love what has changed and what has remained the same in the cosmetic world.

I live, now, where not many care for shopping; people prefer living in their shorts and bathing suits, flip-flops and crocs. Makeup on faces rarely exists, replaced by sunscreen and chap-stick. I love my different existence now. Even shopping at the grocery store is, by comparison to cities, laughably casual. Sometimes I even see people pushing carts in their bathing suits with a cover-up or tee shirt over them. No one cares; that's life in the small village where I live a bohemian life in comparison to busy metros.

For too many years, I dressed 'to the nines', as the saying goes. My job in the cosmetic industry required high heeled shoes to be worn on marble floors. For eight hours, females in the industry stood on heels of terrifying heights, dressed like they were going to a cocktail party. Hair perfectly coiffed, jewelry on every arm and finger and throat and ear. Finally, somewhere in the eighties, uniforms became mandatory for most workers. Every company had designer coats or smocks for ladies behind the counter. There was the aqua blue of the Estée Lauder team, the pink and grey of the Lancôme gals. The Borghese beauties wore black with touches of red depending on the year. Styles came and went. Iconic Chanel was always black and white with touches of gold and the Clinique ladies were all in laboratory white. Varieties of these colors were scattered across the other brands. I thought one day that it seemed like these ladies were beautiful, caged birds of every feather sequestered behind the confines of their cubicles. The employees were happy about the uniforms; wearing them saved their own clothes from wear and tear and lessened cleaning bills. Soon, women behind the counters begged to be allowed to wear more comfortable shoes; so, flats and low-heeled wedges were allowed. But the makeup artists who worked solely for the company, not the department stores or boutique shops, were still required to wear the high heels. Many of us, myself included, suffer the consequences of that edict to this day.

As I sit by the sea outside our front door, I try to focus on those euphoric times. Working in the cosmetic industry for twenty years, my memories were of kind days, fond times within the departments of thriving stores. Hard work, to be sure. But friendships made, sometimes for life.

Lately, I was remembering stories that needed to be journaled so as to never forget. Customers who were sometimes delightful, other times outrageously pompous and condescending. But overall, experiencing the joy of transforming ladies into better versions of themselves. Watching the thrill on their faces as they recognized how attractive they could become with just a few tips on skincare and makeup application. Seeing customers, who now became friends, as they popped by to see what was new and ask what I thought of a particular color or technique.

Most of the time, it was a job one could love. I began as a free-lance makeup artist for about five years. I worked for every brand in the store. Then a prestigious company hired me as a rotating artist where I traveled my city working in all the malls exclusively for that amazing company. Finally, I was tapped as an assistant to the National makeup artist traveling to many cities in the eastern part of the U.S. I loved it and had found my calling.

Then there were other times when certain events happened that could be frightening, scary even. Or shocking. Or uproariously comical. I'll take this time to remember and to pass on to you, the reader, the life of cosmetic queens, makeup artists to the public across much of America. You'll hear opinions on what is sold as miracle creams and oils, what works and what doesn't; what to avoid and what is worth purchasing at any price.

This is a little book for ladies, and lucky for them, for the men who care enough, love them enough, to be aware of what it takes to be a woman in a beauty-obsessed world.

CHAPTER TWO

It's the eighties. The era of big hair, shoulder pads and free thinkers. And lots of makeup. The "natural" look was out, glamour was in. Especially in cities. In the United States, the cities where I've seen the most glamorous, well dressed, well kept, perfectly beautiful women are Dallas, Atlanta and Miami. Of course, New York, but only the upper-class socialites and non-working women fall into the category of perfectly coiffed hair and exquisitely applied makeup. It takes hours, but they make the time. Their husbands require it.

New York is largely businesswomen rushing to offices, hailing cabs and gulping down quick lunches. They are more than likely also mothers who are rushing their children to day-care or schools, then hurrying to work. They are often found in navy or black attire, usually suits, with very little time for creative makeup. Their faces are often fresh washed, devoid of foundation or blush. Perhaps a powdered nose and a slash of pale lipstick is it for the day. Then there are the thousands of young dreamers, students and career chasers who also rush to their destinations. Rushing is the name of the game in the city that never sleeps. These young opportunity seekers never bother with anything on their faces. They usually have long hair, sometimes pulled into a messy ponytail and black is the order of the day for their wardrobes. New York has a look of its own.

Dallas and Atlanta have beautiful women. Beautiful because they just are, and also beautiful for the care they take of themselves. These gals grew up with the same meticulous styling taught to them by their mothers. Maybe it's a hold-over from antebellum days when being southern, or Texas-southern, (and there's a difference) meant always looking your best, knowing how to enhance your looks from an early age. Dallas and Atlanta's women are always bejeweled, a compliment to their husbands who can afford to keep them that way. They care about their wardrobe and have a closet full of fine clothes. Black is big during the day for career women, especially in the cold months. But you can bet there's a gorgeous coat or fur (fake or not) to wrap over the black. (I know a gal who always wore her mink coat to shop for groceries.) But, most importantly, they take great care of their complexions. They've learned over the years what too much sun does to delicate skin. So, they shop constantly for the latest and greatest remedy for lines and wrinkles. Their budget for skin care is usually enormous. They visit salons and cosmetic counters regularly for makeovers, learning the latest techniques to bring out eye color or where to place blush on cheekbones. Southern women have an 'elan' exclusively theirs.

Then there's Miami. That sexy city has a look like no other. The women in tropical Miami and most cities in south Florida really know how to flaunt glamor. Most are of Latin descent and love lots of hair, tons of jewelry, and glorious clothes. They have magnificent, smooth skin and seem ageless. They dress provocatively in the evening and even alluring during the day. To watch a Miami Latina walk across the street is to be treated to a peacock doing a dance of desire. "Look at me, look at me," she seems to be saying. And she loves all the attention. But Miami girls, 'chicas', are also fun and ready for a party. They relish their figures and take advantage of the fact that they are slim and curvaceous in their early years. But even matrons sporting a few extra pounds don't care. They strut like their daughters and never seem to stop smiling. Needless to say, Miami ladies love their makeup. The cosmetic counters in Miami malls ring up sales to equal those in New York. Add to this the fact that well-heeled South Americans make scheduled trips to Miami to stock up on beauty products. It is nothing for favorite counters to be completely bare of product after these ladies have blown through town. I once sold out of every lipstick color in stock for one shopper to take home. One shopper. Thousands of dollars. There was not a tube left.

Ahh, the Latinas of Miami. Especially Puerto Rican girls. They dress scantily and walk like they're on a runway at a fashion show. They are a lot of fun when they hit the cosmetic department. They attack every counter and buy the latest in skin care and color. They are magnificent. Especially because they usually choose to speak English to a gringa like me.

I had a unique experience one day when an Arab Sheik and his entourage approached my counter. The graceful woman beside the Sheik was dressed entirely in a black burka. Even her eyes were covered. She spoke not a word, withdrawing one elegant hand from her sleeve and pointing to the products she wished to purchase. She whispered to her husband the products she desired. One red tipped finger designated the item. As they walked slowly around the counter, I glimpsed a slender ankle bejeweled in golden ankle bracelets. Red toenails, high heeled mules. For her husband's eyes only. They spent thousands, then moved on to other counters.

CHAPTER THREE

But back to the eighties. Discos were still alive and well but were about to be a thing of the past. Girls in the cosmetic departments in nearly every large city shed their required uniforms at the end of the day, having worn something exciting underneath. They visited nightspots all across the city in groups of two to five. The next day, usually a Saturday, many were tired and it showed on their faces. They knew exactly what to do. In the ladies' room, they held cold water compresses under their eyes, then raided the counters for eye creams and concealers. But by ten o'clock when the stores opened, they looked refreshed and ready to sell amazing products.

A really fool-proof eye treatment, although there are many, proved to be a favorite for employees and customers alike. It still is. Shiseido, the oldest cosmetic company in the world, has a sure-fire product for under eyes. Its cream discourages wrinkling and helps with puffiness. It sells out like gang-busters. Shiseido, the inventor of toothpaste, is an international Japanese cosmetics company. Shiseido is excellent skin care but perhaps their star is the eye cream. They also own other lines, among them Drunk Elephant which is a hoot of a name. I buy it just for the name!

One young employee who had just started working in one of my stores was a beauty I'll call Marlene. She was a striking redhead with luminous skin. She was a high school graduate from a small town in the south. Marlene had always known that she wanted to do other people's make-up. She landed a job in a busy department store in a high-end mall. She loved her job, but she *really* loved living in the big city. She quickly learned where all the best live music, bars and clubs were. Every evening after work, she began visiting them, either with girl friends or alone. She started coming to work a little later everyday. Some days she never showed up at all, calling-in to say she was running a fever. Marlene had frequent warnings, but tearfully, she always found forgiveness and got another chance. Still, she just couldn't stay in her rental apartment at night by herself. She became a regular at all the hip places. After her warning, she came to work faithfully, smelling faintly of gin. She clocked in on the mandatory timecard; it verified that she was, indeed, at work.

But Marlene somehow showed up at her counter after lunch. No one noticed at first; it was assumed that she was working the evening shift. Then one day, a customer looking for a dressing room to try on outfits discovered Marlene asleep on the floor. Turns out she'd been getting away with this trick for weeks. Bleary eyed, she knew there would be no more chances. She was fired forever, and people saw her buying a bus ticket back to her small town.

Many a cosmetic consultant had the wrong idea about the job before they started. They figured it was all fun and making people beautiful.... "Painting faces" as the saying goes. They envisioned being able to take home all manner of samples and old testers. They didn't count on the aching legs and feet, how their back hurt after standing up for eight hours with only a lunch break—sometimes a mere 30 minutes. Nor did they realize the tensions and arguing that can arise among the girls who share the counter.

Every week, certain catfights erupted, usually over who should get a sale. If one girl began to aid a customer, but another interfered with the sale, there was always the question of who should be credited with making the sale. Department managers and company executives kept close attention to each employee's results, often giving them a quota. This produced jealousy and resentment to some extent or another almost constantly. Many went home in tears on more than one occasion.

The best cosmetic departments to work in are, ironically, also the worst. High end stores like Neiman Marcus and Saks employ workers on a commission basis only. There is no salary, but the commission rate is adequate-usually nine to ten percent of the sale. Good income is the reward because an employee can sell anything in the entire store for commission. If a customer comes to a cosmetic counter to buy products, an astute associate will find out where she plans to shop next in the store. Accordingly, they will walk the shopper to the next department and show her jewelry, mink coats, purses, shoes, whatever she's looking for. The happy employee gets a percent of everything her 'new best friend' customer buys. Take-home pay can be substantial.

But then there's the other side of this system. As you can imagine, the competition is fierce. Fights over sales can be vicious. I knew one gal that had an on-going feud with her counter mate. One day it came to a head and, in an argument over who should get the sale, my friend had her fingers badly cut when her rival slammed the cash register drawer on them. Another time, two girls were battling it out over who should have gotten credit for an enormous sale. The confrontation spilled out into the floor of the department, then into the main store among the multitude of shoppers. Short of slugging each other, the fight ended when one girl picked up a faux ficus tree out of its container and started beating her rival with it. Ultimately, both were asked to leave their positions and never come back.

These types of high-end stores carry only the best cosmetic lines. The employees are sent to a training school for each company so they can be experts on all aspects of each product. My ultimate favorite is a product line that few can afford. La Prairie has been around for decades but is considered the 'taj mahal' of companies. Their moisturizers can cost over seven hundred dollars for a single jar. If one purchases everything for a skin care regimen from this brand, the bill will be in the thousands of dollars. But the products are incredible. They do exactly what they say they will do. La Prairie is a Swiss company who manufactures skin care from sheep placenta. The cells gleaned from these membranes are as close to human skin as possible. Results are amazing. A new line is Noble Panacea, which is on the order of LaPrairie and is pricey as well.

More than in any other area where people spend money, in cosmetics you get what you pay for. If you go too inexpensive, you won't get the results you're looking for. And, in some cases, you may be adversely affected by a product with cheap ingredients. Of course, some women are just born with fabulous skin and have genetics that make their complexion ageless. I once had a customer who had that lovely, olive-skinned coloring that Spanish and Italian women have. She told me that she used only Crisco to moisturize her skin. Crisco! But miraculously, she had no clogged pours, pimples or blackheads. Just smooth, unwrinkled skin. Her eyelashes were also thick and long. This woman was not young-somewhere in her sixties. Her secret for her lush lashes? Olive oil. So, some people don't have to worry too much about what to put on their face. However, the majority of us don't fall into that category and need to pay attention to what we use on our complexions (and all-over skin, too; but that's a conversation for another day.)

That being said, doing anything is better than doing nothing. I know people who never wash their face. They go to bed with make-up on and never use moisturizer. By their forties, they have rough, wrinkled skin and look twenty years older.

Even drugstore products are better than doing nothing. As far as cleansing is concerned, avoid washing with soap. Use a gentle cleanser like a cream, lotion or alcohol-free gel. L'Oréal, sister company of Lancôme, is a good choice for those on a budget. They have a nice cleanser, then follow with an alcohol-free toner. (Unless you're very oily, then use one with a little alcohol.) People don't understand toner, but it is essential if you want optimum results. It removes any residue from cleansing and Ph balances the skin. It prepares your face for the next step-- moisturizer and eye cream.

There are a lot of 'serums' out now which are mainly for the aging baby-boomer population. As skin dries out and wrinkles, a super concentrated dose of moisture with all kinds of miracle items added is called for. Most have hyaluronic acid, the miracle helper for all skin types. Some have stem cells and collagen. These serums are usually at the top of the scale as far as cost goes. If you're young, you can forgo these for awhile.

Back to drugstore talk. I like most all the L'Oréal products, a fair-priced line. I also like Neutrogena. Try to buy a small amount of any product to try at first. See if you have breakouts or reactions to these inexpensive products. Avoid highly fragranced lotions and creams. This also applies to the higher priced products. If they smell too perfumed, do not purchase. One moisturizer of a medium-priced department store brand is returned on a regular basis due to people getting reactions, usually headaches, from the smell.

Recently, Ulta and Sephora have tried to make shopping for cosmetics easier. They have created a mini store that is supposed to condense down the cosmetic departments of the large stores. It has worked. Sort of. These two do not have nearly the variety of brands offered in mainstream stores, especially the high-end lines. But they do have rows and rows of color products, mostly on the budget end. Teenagers love them and that's okay as these establishments cater to the young and hip. But if you need serious skincare help, these are not for you. Often, I have shopped there for awhile without ever being approached by a helpful worker. It's up to you to fend for yourself. And every time I purchase, I'm in shock at the prices. No deals here. And they are reluctant, in my opinion, to refund my money if I'm unhappy.

Speaking of returns, most people assume cosmetic packages and jars, once opened, cannot be returned for a refund. You may be pleasantly surprised. Be sure to ask at the counter what their policy is. One legendary department store in the South *always* accepted returns, no matter the reason. When I worked in the store, they cheerfully took back jars of moisturizers that were almost empty. The customer would say it broke her out. No questions asked, she was given a refund. Half-used tubes of lipstick, nearly empty mascaras, eye shadows that had holes in the center. This store had drawers full of returned items. It was company policy- the "customer was always right." Seriously, especially if you have sensitive skin, always ask about the ability to bring a product back. Purchasing online is more popular than ever, but you rarely can return, especially if it's coming from overseas.

These days, the latest craze are nice primers you can buy retail or order on line that are applied with a sponge. These are wonderful for a barely-there look or under foundation.

Lipstick is one of my favorite things. I always wore pale, conservative colors until I began to work for a company that was famous for red lips. I applied it one day and went into shock. But gradually, I realized it brought out my eye color. I started getting compliments. So be brave and experiment with shades that are new to you. Ask your BFF what she thinks. A true BFF will always tell you the truth. Again, this is where you can save money. Several high-end companies charge over sixty dollars for a tube of their lipstick. The colors are dazzling, but really? I love the old stand-by of Revlon lipstick. It stays on well, moisturizing the lips without 'bleeding.' As for red lips, Taylor Swift has brought attention to the array of reds in her repertoire and those colors are flying off the shelves.

You can also save on mascara, eyeliner and brow products at drugstores and the like. They're fine for everyday. But for glamor at night and special events, spring for one of the pricier brands. They do indeed have a more polished look to them. Have the make-up artists at the counter show you how to apply these chic looks so you can feel you got your money's worth. One cosmetic brand famous for it's signature look is Chanel. I can spot someone wearing the unique Chanel look every time. And we're not talking about the iconic clothes we all wish we could afford. I mean the smooth, finished look of the face when one has the complete Chanel look. The same is true for Giorgio Armani products. Their foundation gives a luminous, dewy look that turns heads.

As for foundation, whether it's a light, natural look or more coverage, it should always be matched *to your skin on your neck, or throat.* A big taboo are the ladies that have a line between their face and their neck. No blending will take care of that. If you want a tan look, don't get it from foundation.

Get it from bronzing powder, blush stick or a deeper shade of powder than your foundation.

Chanel Beaute,' as their cosmetic line is called, is as fine a product as the exquisite clothes are from the House of Chanel. And the cosmetic branch of the company strives to be just as elegant and sophisticated as the fashion side of the business. The same goes for Dior. The two companies are not related except that they originated in Paris and share a warehouse. You will never see the employees of Chanel or Dior hawking in the aisles of a department store, trying to hook a customer. They are always ready to supply a sample of a particular item, but there will never be specials and gifts to lure customers. They pride themselves on their reputation and know the buying public will seek them out, not the other way around.

Estée Lauder is a leader in the market and is the second biggest conglomerate in the industry. People flock to their counters largely due to their fairly priced inventory. In my opinion, they fall in the 'middle' ratings of cosmetics, along with Borghese and Lancôme. Their products are nice but a lot of them have a lot of fragrance. Their colors are very bold and can sometimes be garish. Use caution when applying. They are by no means up to the quality of La Prairie, Chanel, Dior, Sisley, Armani or some of the high-end lines. Sisley is renowned for their sun-care line. There is none better. Estée Lauder is right there with Lancôme and Clinique as far as middle priced and middle quality lines. In fact, Clinique is owned by Estée Lauder and is considered their more pure, even organic, line. Clinique, to my mind, is made for younger people, especially teenagers or those with problem skin. I would never tell a mature woman who is looking to improve aging to purchase Clinique. Estée Lauder also owns MAC, Tom Ford beauty, LaMer and more. All of these are medium priced and budget worthy. I love LaMer best of all these companies, in fact, they are possibly up there with the top lines as far as results are concerned.

Doctors are lending their names now to skin care because of the lucrative income from them. Obagi and Skin Medica are my favorites and have very little fragrance. Again, you get what you pay for, so that goes for dermatological brands as well. In my mind, they are mid-range as far as results.

But visiting a dermatological office is a must-do. They check for skin cancers and can offer laser and micro-peel treatments that really help with pore size and sun damage. Have as many of these as you can afford.

As for Botox and the like, that's up to you. But choose a clinic or doctor after you've seen results on a friend or two. Don't fall for ads and specials. The proof is in the pudding by seeing actual clients. A very well-known and excellent dermatologist may still not be the best for injections and treatments. My friend loved her dermatologist until he injected her with Dysport (like Botox), hit a nerve and caused the client to have a sagging eyelid for nearly a year. Ask questions of friends who have had good experiences *consistently*.

While we're discussing Botox, Dysport and the like, of course the rage in facial enhancers is fillers. In lips, cheeks, chins, etc. products like Juvéderm and Radiesse have good results, but again, choose a clinician that has given your friends good outcomes. Fillers don't last forever, any where from six months to two years. And unlike what some providers will tell you, they don't just dissolve. They actually move. So, take care and be cautious. More and more, role models in movies and television are opting to age naturally and do minimal enhancement. (We've all seen pictures of the freaky results on some of these once-beautiful people.)

The same thing applies to face-lift surgery. Study results on some of your friends and choose very cautiously. Interview several doctors and look at their result pictures.

Check their board certification. Remember they don't show the pictures of clients who may be unhappy. Again, search out friends and acquaintances who are happy with their outcomes. By the way, always have good facials as much as you can. The cosmetic counters are not set up to give adequate facials, so find a good esthetician and pamper yourself. Always use a mask (exfoliation or hydrating) at home between facials.

A lot of gals in the cosmetic industry shave. Yes, really. Shaving is a sort of 'planing'-all the rage now. It removes dead skin cells and facial hair so you get a fresh, polished look with or without makeup. (Caution: if you happen to have dark facial hair instead of peach fuzz, better to have a professional esthetician remove it with waxing or laser.)

Remember what was said before— doing *anything* is better than doing nothing. All cosmetic companies manufacture their products to be used as a *whole.* Each step in skin care is designed to work together with the next step in the line. This probably brings the best results. But if you like the eye cream of one line and the moisturizer of another, feel free to buy what you like. Especially in the color lines, if you like the eyeshadows of Lancôme and the lipstick of Dior, go ahead and mix it up.

Try to have a shopping day once a year for skincare and beauty products. Or let it be the Christmas present you ask for. Husbands and boyfriends come sheepishly to the counters around Christmas or birthday time. He knows only that the woman in his life likes a certain product. It eases his mind and makes it all simple when a lovely basket is filled with products, shrink-wrapped and tied with a beautiful bow. And his lady will think he hung the moon.

Speaking of Christmas, working in a cosmetic department during the Christmas holiday is both exciting and taxing. Starting right after, and sometimes even before Halloween, out come the decorations. The display department has so much to do, they start decorating beauty departments first. Long before Thanksgiving, Christmas songs and carols are piped in, ringing all over the store. The atmosphere is exhilarating at first; but by Christmas it is mind-boggling and exhausting. The noise level in these departments can rise to deafening heights. Driving home, I couldn't bear to hear even a radio. One evening after weeks of the Christmas build-up, my husband wanted to take me to dinner. When I got to the restaurant, I turned right around. I couldn't go in, couldn't stand anymore loudness. It was definitely noise overload. I just wanted quiet for the rest of the year. As beautiful as it is in the store, we long to get back to the plain old everyday routine.

Mothers and daughters can have a rewarding and bonding experience when mom brings her teenager for a tutorial on skincare. Basic products can be purchased. The fun part is letting the budding beauty opt for some color choices. But you don't have to be like the well-heeled mother who brought her 11-year-old to our counter in south Florida when I was there. Her daughter was polite but basically uninterested even though her mom dropped 2500 dollars on goodies for her child. A little extreme.

CHAPTER FOUR

Ah, love. Whenever you have women working together day after day in close quarters, you hear about the good, the bad and the ugly of their love lives. Most females understand the ups and downs of relationships and offer a listening ear and shoulder to cry on. The support of her fellow divas at work has gotten many a gal through rough times in the love department.

While I worked in my home store between traveling for cosmetic events, a friend and counter- mate fell in love. But it was a strange romance.

The telephone at our counter, a vital lifeline for customers to call in and order products, was on the fritz. It wouldn't ring and we couldn't call out. A telephone technician was called in to resolve the problem; he and my friend Rosalie struck up a conversation. The phone worked for a few days, then died again. Back came Earl, the same guy, to fix it again. This time, he took his time. More conversation with Rosalie, less attention to the dead phone. But he got it working again. By third time it gave out, he seemed to be a regular at the counter. He and Rosalie exchanged numbers and after a while, an affair ensued.

Turns out, Earl was married and lived at least ninety minutes from his job. He drove that distance every day. He was at his job, then spent time with Rosalie in the evenings.

By the time he arrived back at home, it was very late at night. Rosalie was so in love with Earl she seemed to float into work each day. She blushed with the glow of love. She was a lovely platinum blonde with exquisite skin and deep brown eyes. Her eyelashes were enhanced a bit but she was expert at this. Even we makeup girls couldn't tell. She was a little bit of a 'chubbette' with hips that filled up most of the space behind the counter. But a real beauty. Earl seemed head-over-heels when he visited. Rosalie was sure he would leave his wife and marry her. We weren't as convinced.

One day, I came to work early and Rosalie and I were the only two in our cubicle. Soon, two women approached the counter but were not smiling. They asked me, "are you Rosalie?" I answered no but said, "this is Rosalie right over there." Rosalie happily approached them. The shorter of the two women suddenly raised her voice. "You slut! You are having an affair with my husband and I'm gonna tell you it's gonna stop! We have children and he will never give up his family for you, you whore!" The color drained from Rosalie's face as she stepped back. She was speechless. She started to shake. Then the assailant opened her purse and there lay a black pistol. "I'm gonna stop this right now!" Said Earl's wife.

Rosalie was in shock. For some reason, I stepped in front of Rosalie and glared at the women. I threw my arms out to protect Rosalie. I yelled at the gun-toting hussy, "you get outta here right now. Back off. I'm calling security!" Just then, an angel in disguise in the form of a security guard was walking in the aisle near our counter. I called to him that we had a problem. As he rushed over, the two females ran for the door and he gave chase. I never knew what happened after that.

Rosalie sank to the floor behind the counter, crumbling into hysterics. "I'm not givin' him up!" She cried. She was trembling as I tried to help her to stand. Finally, it took three of us to get her up. The incident was the talk of the department for days. It frightened all of us. Nowadays, there are metal detectors in many mall stores in big cities, but in the late eighties that was not the case.

The story of Rosalie and Earl had an unhappy ending. Their affair continued for several more months; Earl said he had retained an attorney in his small town. Then one night, after being with Rosalie until the wee hours, Earl was driving the ninety miles back home when he fell asleep. His truck careened off the highway down a cliff. He was killed instantly. Rosalie was never the same after that. All her plans and dreams had died that night with Earl. She rarely smiled. She seemed so alone. Then she adopted a cat and retreated into herself even more.

But not all love stories ended so sadly. Beautiful flowers frequently arrived at the counters from some lothario. Once, a soldier who was in love with an Estée Lauder girl showed up unexpectedly and got down on one knee after he brought her out from behind the counter. He proposed, produced a lovely ring and she said yes. The whole department, employees and customers, burst into applause and tears.

Once when I was working with the national makeup artist in Tampa, a young gal who worked for Clinique came in with a black eye. It took the skills of all of us to conceal it. Her fellow employees knew she was in an abusive relationship. She often came to her job in tears but was afraid to leave him because she had a child. On this particular day, her friends in the department took charge. With help from the kind department manager, she was taken to a women's refuge where she was able to live with her toddler. The amazing store provided her a 'leave of absence' and she received her regular paycheck until she found a place of her own. She found the courage to call the police to arrest the partner that had beaten her. So, there was a happy ending to this story, one of many in the world of cosmetic-dom.

Another saga in the search for love is the story of Peter. Peter was a familiar face to all the ladies who worked in cosmetics in many stores in the large mall. He was a tenured professor of literature at a well-known university. He spoke with a British accent and was impeccably dressed. With his white, brushed back hair and his six-foot two stature, he turned a lot of heads. Most of us found him delightfully attractive. He tried to date a lot of girls and invited many of us to join him to dine on our lunch hour. He seemed not interested in a relationship; he just loved spending time with a beautiful lady.

One such beautiful lady was Judith. She was fair skinned with a mane of dark brunette hair and hazel eyes. She was petite with a stunning figure. She was married but just seemed happy to enjoy Peter's company. She was one of his favorite lunch partners. One day in mid week, Peter was wandering around the department, talking to several ladies. He ended up at Judith's counter for the appointed lunch date. Off they went to the elegant dining room in the department store. It served delicious food and was a favorite of employees and shoppers alike.

Peter and Judith sat a secluded table where they could talk. Peter ordered the special and Judith decided on a nourishing vegetable soup. It was delicious because it had a lot of herbs and spices. In the middle of their conversation, Judith began to cough. Then she started a sort of choking. She had swallowed a large bay leaf that had not been scooped out of the soup. It was lodged over her windpipe. She choked louder, turning red. Peter, discreet gentleman that he was, did not wish to embarrass Judith; so he looked away, pretending not to pay attention to her predicament. Judith began to feel she couldn't breathe. She beat on her chest. Peter still ignored the situation in his perfectly appropriate way, just as he had been taught. Then Judith fell from her chair in a faint on the carpet beside the table. At last, Peter realized something was wrong. He knelt beside her, gently tapping on her back. Waiters and managers rushed to her aid; finally, paramedics were called. They tended to Judith while Peter patted her hand. Determined to return to her counter, Judith, escorted by Peter, finished her workday with a smile and quite a tale.

Men just love cosmetic departments. There were always fellows walking up and down the aisles around the counters. Every now and then, they'd wander up to a certain lady and make small talk about the products. Then they would get around to finding out if she had a husband or a boyfriend. Most were just regarded as a nuisance, interfering in a workday. But sometimes, real romances started.

One time, there was a bomb threat at Neiman's and the store had to be evacuated. It turned out to be a hoax, but a multitude of policemen stayed for hours inspecting every store. When they came into our store, they kind of delayed when they were inspecting the cosmetic section. A cute cop named Greg struck up a conversation with my friend Donna. He was absolutely entranced by the pert blonde with the big smile. He found a reason to visit day after day. One small detail—Donna already had a husband, but she didn't like him very much. In short order, she dumped husband number one. Then Greg began offering Donna a lift home. This went on for some months. One day, Donna came to work with a ring on her finger. They were married soon after.

The story of Greg and Donna has an odd ending. For some reason, Greg was either fired or resigned from the police department. He looked for another job. So in love were they, that Donna begged for Greg to find a job that she could share with him. The last we heard, he landed a gig as a cross-country trucker and Donna accompanied him on every trip. I can just imagine it.

CHAPTER FIVE

Men. As stated before, men love to pass by the cosmetic department at mall stores. They are usually polite and try not to be obvious about the stares. It doesn't bother the employees much, as long as these men keep their distance. If one of them enters into the counter Mecca, all eyes are on him and there are lots of ladies who come to help the potential buyer. Usually, he is buying a gift for a wife or daughter or sweetheart. And men seem clueless about what cosmetics and fragrances really cost. Often, they are surprised but whip out a credit card anyway. He loves it if the gifts are prettily wrapped and appreciates added samples of lotions and perfumes. He really likes it if some of the colognes are for males.

Sometimes, men who hang around seem creepy. Almost every lady who works in the department knows how to spot a creep. They have a certain look, a definite demeanor. Often, security is asked to hover nearby just in case the creep tries to approach. In the last years of working in malls, I requested security to provide a guard to walk me to my car. It was during that time that an incident happened that is both funny and frightening.

Most everyone in cosmetic-dom knew Carla. She was a statuesque beauty who worked in cosmetics at Neiman Marcus. A woman of color, she wore her dark hair pulled into a tight bun. She had perfect, caramel colored skin and amber eyes. She was an asset to the store. One night she worked late and, when it was time to leave, she declined the company of a security officer to walk her to her car. She walked out into the darkness and down to her vehicle. A man stood in her way as she approached. He wore a hat pulled down over his eyes and a raincoat. She stopped in her tracks. Then he opened his raincoat. He was stark naked. I don't know what kind of shock reaction he expected from his victim, but he had picked the wrong girl. "Hmmm," said Carla, unperturbed. Cool as a cucumber, she said, "Looks like a ______, only smaller." The perpetrator slunk away back into the shadows like the coward he was. When all the girls heard about it, all they could say was, "you go girl!"

Some men come to a counter to have *their own* makeup done. Some seem genuinely interested in skin care for themselves. Men can now have their makeup done openly but years ago, that caused too much of a stir; so they were taken to a private room to have it applied.

I remember two women who came to have their makeup done. I worked with one lady while my counter-mate beautified the other. They were dressed beautifully, had amazing hair and nice skin. About half-way through the session, I noticed my lady had a rather large Adam's apple. About that time, I also noticed a five-o'clock shadow. My partner eyed me with a knowing look. I gave her a wink and we realized we were working on two cross-dressing men. When the appointment ended, both women looked stunning. They purchased all the products we recommended and went their happy way.

But one day a gentleman came up to the counter, very shy and reticent. He was dressed in a business suit and tie. Nice looking, seemed like he might be a lawyer or something. He didn't say a word, just handed me a note. It was in a small envelope. I opened it and saw a yellow and blue design on the note that turned out to be little ducks in a row. Very delicate. In a woman's handwriting, the note said, "My husband enjoys wearing makeup, eyeshadow and lipstick. This is fine with me. Please give him a nice evening look." I asked the department manager what she thought about him sitting at the counter while I did his makeup. She flatly refused but said we could take him to a private room. When I told him this, he got tears in his eyes and raced out the door. Never dull in cosmetic departments.

CHAPTER SIX

By the mid-nineties, and up until today, the industry started to change. More males were applying to work in cosmetics. All of them were gay. They were funny and a joy to work with, for the most part. Customers seemed to love them. Gay men are usually very creative and absolutely love the opportunity to work in an artistic industry with women. Soon, it seemed my generation of women were seen less and less in the industry.

I had worked and traveled with the national makeup artist for our company. A gay man himself, he was charming and a creative genius. He was tall and very good looking. He turned heads of both sexes everywhere he went. Whenever he was booked for special events on the east coast of the U.S., he requested that I be his assistant. For some reason, he just loved me and respected my ability to relate to customers and sell. We had a merry time together, traveling to some exciting cities with our rep, me and the famed Eduardo. It was exciting to be in his company and pick up tips from him. Eduardo was Cuban by birth, but his family migrated to Texas after they came to America. Clients probably assumed he was gay, but they fell for him anyway when he looked deeply into their eyes while he made them beautiful. He lightly touched their skin, held their chins in his strong hand when he was adding eyeshadow and liner. They were enchanted. He had a way with women for sure. They would have bought anything he suggested and usually did. The end result was extraordinary sales for each store he visited.

Eduardo graced my home store about once a year. He had just finished his four days at our counter performing miracles for delighted customers. He flew out that night. We were all exhausted in a happy, rewarding kind of way. The next morning, I arrived early at work, walking into the department with the first of the counter girls on the morning shift. We were just settling in, organizing the counters, chatting brightly. Suddenly, renegades wearing all white with what appeared to be blood smeared on their clothes burst into the store, heading straight for the cosmetic department. They ranted and raged, yelling about testing on animals. They carried buckets of what looked like blood (turned out to be paint), as they raced like mad monsters to every counter. They threw the awful red liquid on all the counters, taking direct aim at a few brands. They broke the glass on a few counters, the shards flying everywhere. It took security what seemed like forever to arrive, guns drawn. They chased the intruders out into the mall. Most of us cowered on the floor behind the counters. In tears, we began to clean up the mess. The department was roped off from shoppers until everything was back in order. Protesting was the order of the day. Some cosmetic companies tested a few products, mostly on rats. But ours was not one of them. Now I believe that practice is a thing of the past.

By the end of the nineties, I was not far from retirement. My legs hurt constantly, and I had plantar fasciitis in the soles of my feet. Walking out of a store in the evening was becoming more of a concern. Even in my home store when I wasn't traveling, I had to be escorted to my car each evening by a security guard. Things weren't safe anymore. I'd had three cars stolen from that mall in the last five years of working there. Society in general was becoming more violent. When my husband was offered a job in Florida, I decided it was time to retire. The last day I worked, I cried all day as I left friends and memories behind.

****

In the scriptures, in the book of Genesis, the Hebrew translation of Adams' words when he first saw Eve was the equivalent of "*wow!*" Let that be the mantra by which you live. Always be a 'wow' for your husband, your family. *Yourself.* Take care of yourself and your skin.

But as my mother used to say, “pretty is as pretty does.” Inner beauty is always the most important thing. You can be both.

PLEASE REVIEW

Thank you for reading this book. If you would kindly leave a review on Amazon, I would appreciate it.

www.ingramcontent.com/pod-product-compliance
Lightning Source LLC
LaVergne TN
LVHW022315200926
848481LV00004B/1355
9798349360053